Hanzade Dogan

MIS-UN-TRUE Informed Consent

AF136177

Hanzade Dogan

MIS-UN-TRUE Informed Consent

Focus on informed consent and ethical requirements for clinical trials of neuroscience and psychiatry

LAP LAMBERT Academic Publishing

Impressum / Imprint

Bibliografische Information der Deutschen Nationalbibliothek: Die Deutsche Nationalbibliothek verzeichnet diese Publikation in der Deutschen Nationalbibliografie; detaillierte bibliografische Daten sind im Internet über http://dnb.d-nb.de abrufbar.

Bibliographic information published by the Deutsche Nationalbibliothek: The Deutsche Nationalbibliothek lists this publication in the Deutsche Nationalbibliografie; detailed bibliographic data are available in the Internet at http://dnb.d-nb.de.

Coverbild / Cover image: www.ingimage.com

Verlag / Publisher:
LAP LAMBERT Academic Publishing
ist ein Imprint der / is a trademark of
OmniScriptum GmbH & Co. KG
Heinrich-Böcking-Str. 6-8, 66121 Saarbrücken, Deutschland / Germany
Email: info@lap-publishing.com

Herstellung: siehe letzte Seite /
Printed at: see last page
ISBN: 978-3-659-81428-0

MIS – UN –TRUE INFORMED CONSENT

Focus on informed consent and ethical requirements for clinical trials of neuroscience and psychiatry
A small study and a brief report from Istanbul, Turkey

Hanzade Dogan

Foreword

I have worked on this book not only for medical students but also medical professionals, Institutional Review Board (IRB) members, clinical ethics committee members or patients.

The aim of this work was to reveal the ethical requirements and the quality of informed consent especially for clinical trials in neuroscience.
Focusing on the review of published examples in literature, presentations in relevant meetings, an original small study reflecting the attitudes of healthy volunteers to clinical trials in Istanbul, Turkey.

Ethics is the essence of medicine. Many disciplines of medicine are naturally very close to ethics or in other words they have overlapping topics in decision making, in protocol preparing, education or case analysis. I wanted to emphasize all the methodological overlapping points of those disciplines to contribute to the better application of clinical trials - focusing specifically in neuroscience.

New applications in medicine, psychiatry, neuroscience and technology are changing our lives. Currently, the delicate border between clinical trials and conventional diagnostic / treatment methods is becoming more evident. At this delicate border, while current debate is continuing about novel research techniques, new ethical questions arise, that need both rational and humanistic answers and that affect mankind's understanding of self. What are our responsibilities towards human subjects in clinical trials? What are our responsibilities towards vulnerable psychiatry patients? What are the norms about the routine techniques on minor neurology patients? What are the economic incentives affecting decisions? What are the unethical characteristics about mental health professionals and clinical trials? What makes a clinical research ethical?

Most researchers and clinicians enter the field to help others, satisfy their scientific curiosity, and to make progress, but clinical practice and research endeavors often involve decision-making in the context of ethical ambiguity. Good intentions are absolute requirements, but unfortunately not enough, and have to proceed with rational and humanistic decisions, respect for others' values for a successful "**Ethical Conduct**" that is inevitable.

Medicine - especially certain disciplines - cannot proceed without diagnostic methods that are still under investigation or treatment alternatives that are still being searched. Neuroscience and psychiatry are strong examples to those. I wanted to analyze the discrepancies between the applications and ethical concerns.

Ethical concerns would diminish the scientific burden on human subjects.

Current neuroscience research projects are using EEG and other electrophysiological measures such as EEG/ERP, pharmaco-EEG, or other techniques such as fMRI, TMS or PET to answer questions relevant to better care of patients in the future with unknown mechanisms of disease. Those projects are exposed to the ethical problems of the newly used medication, newly used diagnostic techniques, clinical trials implied as conventional treatment methods, or conventional diagnostic or treatment methods on irrelevant patient groups. Although each technique proposes a different research setting and while this process is going on with the enthusiasm of hardworking researchers, we are still concerned about some commonly observed ethical problems such as mis-un-true informed consent, problems of fair subject selection, incentives in trials, etc.

The Ministry of Health of Turkey implemented new legislation on clinical trials and newly established independent ethics committees in 2011. (Institutional Review Boards-IRBs) These independent and multidisciplinary IRBs analyze research projects and make recommendations about them.

The aim of the book is to review the common neuroscience clinical trials focusing more on EEG related and other electrophysiology trials, to discuss the potential ethical problems in clinical trials of neuroscience on human subjects and to discuss application of ethical requirements in practice and the necessity of a network of independent and multidisciplinary IRBs updating concerns and solutions worldwide composed of talented and educated members. Since electrophysiology measures and neuroimaging techniques are progressively more used to aid diagnosis and treatment in psychiatry and other areas of neuroscience, if trials could be designed on ethical grounds that would be of great help both to researchers and patients.

'Mis-Un-True informed consent' is my new terminology for the informed consent process in clinical trials. The terminology does not aim to criticize any process but to enlighten the realities, conditions and values relevant to the process.

Truth is always a friendly guide to choices, ethical processes and medical applications.

Hanzade Dogan
Istanbul, 2016

CONTENTS

ACKNOWLEDGEMENTS

I would highly appreciate Prof. Dr. Kemal Arıkan's cooperative efforts - The Department of Liaison-Consultation Psychiatry- whenever I needed his valuable academic consultation.

Moreover, all his valuable partnership with clinical ethics projects, applications and meetings and his guidance for psychiatric information respecting all the patients and human subjects in principle is of incredible value.

 I am really thankful to him.

INTRODUCTION

Progress and new applications in medicine, psychiatry, neuroscience and technology are changing our lives. The delicate border between clinical trials and conventional diagnostic / treatment methods is becoming more evident. At this delicate border, while current debate is continuing about novel research techniques, new ethical questions arise, that need both rational and humanistic answers and that affect mankind's understanding of self.

Most clinicians and scientists within the triangle of the best service of conventional treatment methods to the best interest of the patients, presentation of the current technological advances and compliance with the curiosity of the experimental methods, are often involved in the decision-making process in the context of ethical ambiguity.

Mental Health Professionals and researchers encounter many ethical questions and dilemmas of informed consent in their everyday practice, research, and teaching. It is expected that, health professionals who are trained to provide the best service to vulnerable groups believe and understand that their service should be embedded in a logical, humanistic and ethical framework.

Guidelines regarding "Research Consenting" such as Nuremberg, Helsinki, Belmont, American Counseling Associates Code of Ethics (2005), American Psychiatry Associates (APA) The Principles of Medical Ethics with Annotations Especially Applicable to Psychiatry (2006) and Legislations of nations about protections of human subjects are well known and widely available. In those guidelines human rights, values are respected and the principles of respect, beneficence and justice are basic elements. However, when it comes to applications and daily practice, there are still lots of ethical concerns of the Institutional Review Boards, patients, public, professionals about the conduct of clinical trials and daily practice. Therefore we should first review what makes applications unethical in general, so that we might further continue our search and discussion in specific areas such as 'clinical trials' involving EEG, other electrophysiology measures, pharmaco-EEG trials and others like neuroimaging etc.

Unethical characteristics of mental health professionals and researchers in general terms

Koecher et al, described very clearly the possible underlying unethical characteristics of mental health professionals and researchers in general terms in their book published in 2008 as follows:

- Are ignorant or misinformed regarding the ethical standards of their profession;
- Practice outside their realm of competence and expertise, with or without awareness;
- Show insensitivity to the needs of those with whom they work or to situational dynamics;
- Exploit clients by putting their own needs first;
- Behave irresponsibly due to laziness, stress, lack of awareness, or other reasons that take their attention away from their professional responsibilities;
- Seek vengeance against perceived harms to themselves by clients or others with whom they work;
- Suffer from burnout or other emotional impairment;
- Have no concept of or have distorted views of interpersonal boundaries;
- Rationalize actions that are often unrecognized as self-serving;
- Usually behave competently, ethically, and with good awareness, but "slip" by losing sight of a goal or becoming momentarily distracted.

Yazıcı quoted in his article:

"A Brief Report from NIH about the trust of public in medicine.....

".....There has been much discussion of late that confidence in medicine is being eroded. No less an authority than Elias A. Zerhouni, M.D., Director of the National Institutes of Health (N.I.H), Bethesda, Maryland, has recently said that forty percent of science news relates to health and medicine and a gradual erosion of public trust is being observed. The main trust of this discussion is the ever profiteering drug industry, the ever loosening professional standards of the physician, and the standing and expectations from the state health authorities, i.e. The Federal Drug Administration (FDA), among others......."

Different settings of Clinical Trials of EEG, electrophysiological measures and pharmaco-EEG trials

Clinical trials of EEG and neuroscience are pre-planned research programs on human subjects to answer specific questions of diagnostic or treatment benefits of EEG and other electrophysiological measures of neuroscience for future patients. Characteristic methods are randomization, blinding, placebo, comparison with control groups, tests for research etc. Justification of risks is the ratio of "value of knowledge to be gained" to "societal benefit". It is important to minimize bias and respect diversity in designing and implementing research. It is different from medical care as the latter is to provide personalized care of psychiatry here and now. Medical care uses individualized and accepted diagnostic and treatment choices. Justification of risks is compensatory direct medical benefit to patient.

Silvana G reports that current debate about the nature of clinical trials of pharmaco-EEG such as it remaining an empirical method in spite of dedication of lots of resources to the subject is continuing. Pharmaco-EEG as a scientific discipline was born with an ambitious goal of providing a scientific method for drug classification alternative to chemical/ pharmacological similarities between substances. However, the trials have some limitations. EEG modifications concomitant to changes such as blood pressure, heart rate, neuro-hormonal status, and alcohol or nicotine level in blood are comparable to those induced by neuroactive compounds. Furthermore, the EEG and its response to drugs depend on the subjects' emotional status, signal baseline prior to administration etc. These point out that because of technical limitations a correct experimental setting and correct management of interactions with human subjects are very important in pharnaco-EEG clinical trials to reduce the variability in electrophysiological changes attributable to drug and large-scale studies have high costs. Silvana et al emphasize that multi-dose, placebo-controlled studies with multiple pre- and post-drug measurements are to be used to compensate for spontaneous or experimentally induced biases. So, pharmaco-EEG clinical trials are not as straight forward as trials of fast developing techniques for functional brain imaging such as TMS, fMRI or NFB.

Common Unethical Characteristics in Clinical Trials of EEG and others in neuroscience

- Lack of "Informed Consent"
- "Uninformed" or "Misinformed" consent
- Impaired risk assessment about newly used measurement techniques, treatment tools and medication.
- Questionable incentives such as "money." especially for healthy subjects.
- Impaired and vulnerable subjects
- Possible impaired settings of clinical trials on patients such as blinding, double blinding, placebo, randomized, invasiveness, expensive etc.
- Difficult settings of pharmaco-EEG trials
- Clinical trials proposed as conventional treatment methods and misinformed or uninformed patient groups

○ Conventional diagnostic methods on irrelevant or misinformed patient groups, etc. for a variety of different reasons and aims.

Electroencephalography (EEG)

Electroencephalography (**EEG**) is the recording of electrical activity along the scalp produced by the firing of neurons within the brain. The main diagnostic application of EEG is in the case of epilepsy, as epileptic activity can create clear abnormalities on a standard EEG study. A secondary clinical use of EEG is in the diagnosis of coma, encephalopathies, and brain death. Although no consensus has been reached, quantified EEG has been proposed to be used in psychiatry to make a diagnosis, and follow up. EEG used to be a first-line method for the diagnosis of tumors, stroke and other focal brain disorders, but this use has decreased with the advent of anatomical imaging techniques such as MRI and CT.

Derivatives of the EEG technique include evoked potentials (EP), which involves averaging the EEG activity time-locked to the presentation of a stimulus of some sort (visual, somatosensory, or auditory). Event-related potentials (ERP) refer to averaged EEG responses that are time-locked to more complex processing of stimuli; this technique is used in cognitive science, cognitive psychology, and psychophysiological research.

Research use of EEG

A different method to study brain function is functional magnetic resonance imaging (fMRI). Some benefits of EEG compared to fMRI include:

- Hardware costs are significantly lower for EEG sensors versus an fMRI machine

- EEG sensors can be deployed into a wider variety of environments than can a bulky, immobile fMRI machine
- EEG enables higher temporal resolution, on the order of milliseconds, rather than seconds
- EEG is relatively tolerant of subject movement versus an fMRI (where the subject must remain completely still)
- EEG is silent, which allows for better study of the responses to auditory stimuli
- EEG does not aggravate claustrophobia

Limitations of EEG as compared with fMRI include:

- Significantly lower spatial resolution
- ERP studies require relatively simple paradigms, compared with block-design fMRI studies

EEG vs. fMRI and PET

EEG has several strong points as a tool for exploring brain activity. EEGs can detect changes within a millisecond timeframe, excellent considering an action potential takes approximately 0.5-130 milliseconds to propagate across a single neuron, depending on the type of neuron. Other methods of looking at brain activity, such as PET and fMRI have time resolution between seconds and minutes. EEG measures the brain's electrical activity directly, while other methods record changes in blood flow (e.g., SPECT, fMRI) or metabolic activity (e.g, PET), which are indirect markers of brain electrical activity. EEG can be used simultaneously with fMRI so that high-temporal-resolution data can be recorded at the same time as high-spatial-resolution data; however, since the data derived from each occurs over a different time course, the data sets do not necessarily represent the exact same brain activity.

Three Examples of relevant published clinical trials from the literature

Example I

Price GW, Lee JN, Garvey CA, Gibson N. The use of background EEG activity to determine stimulus timing as a means of improving rTMS efficacy in the treatment of depression. Brain Stimul. 2010 Jul; 3(3):140-52. Epub 2009 Sep 17. Health Service-Mental Health, Perth, Australia.

Background: Repetitive transcranial magnetic stimulation (rTMS) treatment of depression utilizes numerous predetermined patterns of stimulation. As an alternative to using invariant stimulus timing parameters, the interactive technique delivers individual stimuli based on the background electroencephalogram (EEG) activity.

Objective: This study examines the use of an EEG-dependent technique as a means to enhance the efficacy of rTMS in the treatment of depression.

Methods: Forty-four patients with treatment-refractory major depression were treated, in a randomized, double-blind, 4-week trial, with two different rTMS stimulus timing techniques (left dorsolateral prefrontal cortex). Standard rTMS utilized 10-Hz stimuli, whereas interactive rTMS applied individual stimuli in response to a selected pattern of background EEG activity analyzed in real time. Hamilton Depression Rating Scale (HDRS) and the Beck's Depression Inventory-II (BDI) scores were recorded at baseline, 2 weeks and after the final treatment.

Results: The interactive group showed a trend toward greater efficacy than the standard group in both absolute (t=-1.68; P=.100) and percentage (t=-1.74;

13

P=.090) change in scores on HDRS (and similarly BDI). The response rate (>50% reduction) for the interactive technique of 43% (9/21) was also different to that of the standard technique (22%; 5/23; odds ratio: 2.70).

Conclusion: The use of EEG-based TMS stimuli has been shown to be feasible in an rTMS clinical trial in treatment-resistant depression. The EEG-based interactive technique was associated with an indication of a trend toward a greater clinical effect than the standard rTMS technique. The interactive technique thus has the potential to refine the rTMS methodology and to enhance efficacy in the treatment of depression.

Example II

Kayran S, Dursun e, Dursun N, Ermutlu N, Karamürsel S. Neurofeedback Intervention in Fibromyalgia Syndrome; a Randomized, Controlled, Rater Blind Clinical Trial. Appl Psychophysiol Biofeedback 2010 Jul.

Abstract

We designed a randomized, rater blind study to assess the efficacy of EEG Biofeedback (Neurofeedback-NFB) in patients with fibromyalgia syndrome (FMS). Eighteen patients received twenty sessions of NFB-sensory motor rhythm (SMR) treatment (NFB group) during 4 weeks, and eighteen patients were given 10 mg per day escitalopram treatment (control group) for 8 weeks. Visual Analog Scales for pain and fatigue, Hamilton and Beck Depression and Anxiety Inventory Scales, Fibromyalgia Impact Questionnaire and Short Form 36 were used as outcome measures which were applied at baseline and 2nd, 4th, 8th, 16th, 24th weeks. Mean amplitudes of EEG rhythms (delta, theta, alpha, SMR, beta1 and beta2) and theta/SMR ratio were also measured in NFB group. All post-treatment measurements showed significant improvements in both of the groups (for all parameters $p < 0.05$). NFB group displayed greater benefits than controls (for all parameters p < 0.05). Therapeutic efficacy of NFB was found to begin at 2nd week and reached to a maximum effect at 4th week. On the other hand, the improvements in SSRI treatment were also detected to begin at 2nd week but reached to a maximum effect at 8th week. No statistically significant changes were noted regarding mean amplitudes of EEG rhythms (p > 0.05 for all). However,

theta/SMR ratio showed a significant decrease at 4th week compared to baseline in the NFB group (p < 0.05). These data support the efficacy of NFB as a treatment for pain, psychological symptoms and impaired quality of life associated with fibromyalgia.

This study indicates that NBF procedure cannot be put in the first line treatment procedure.

Example III

LosS, Sobol JB, Mallavaram N, Carsan M, Chang C, Grieve PC, Emerson RC, Stark RI, Sun LS. Anesthetic-specific electroencephalographic patterns during emergence from sevoflurane and isoflurane in infants and children. Pediatr Anaesth 2009 Dec; 19(12): 1157–65.

Background: Devices that monitor the depth of anesthesia are increasingly used to titrate sedation and avoid awareness during anesthesia. Many of these monitors are based upon electroencephalography (EEG) collected from large adult reference populations and not pediatric populations (Anesthesiology, 86, 1997, 836; Journal of Anaesthesia, 92, 2004, 393; Anesthesiology, 99, 2003, 34). We hypothesized that EEG patterns in children would be different from those previously reported in adults and that they would show anesthetic-specific characteristics.

Methods: This prospective observational study was approved by the Institutional Review Board, and informed written consent was obtained. Patients were randomized to receive maintenance anesthesia with isoflurane or sevoflurane. EEG data collection included at least 10 min at steady-state maintenance anesthesia. The EEG was recorded continuously through emergence until after extubation. A mixed model procedure was performed on global and regional power by pooled data analysis and by analyzing each anesthetic group separately. Statistical significance was defined as $P < 0.05$.

Results: Thirty-seven children completed the study (ages 22 days-3.6 years). Isoflurane and sevoflurane had different effects on global and regional EEG power during emergence from anesthesia, and frontal predominance patterns were significantly different between these two anesthetic agents.

Conclusions: The principal finding of the present study was that there are anesthetic-specific and concentration-dependent EEG effects in children. Depth-of-anesthesia monitors that utilize algorithms based on the EEGs of adult reference populations therefore may not be appropriate for use in children.

REVIEWS OF EEG, ELECTROPHYSIOLOGY MEASURES AND NEUROIMAGING RELATED   CLINICAL TRIALS IN NEUROSCIENCE

Currently many clinical trials are being carried out about the diagnostic and treatment potentials of EEG, electrophysiology measures and neuroimaging techniques. Many societies and scientists, technological and pharmacological industry and publishers are in a race of new contributions to the relevant area. Electroencephalography (EEG) and other electrophysiology measures offer the promise of predicting the likelihood that novel therapies and compounds will exhibit clinical efficacy early in preclinical and clinical development. These analyses, including quantitative EEG (e.g. brain mapping), evoked /event- related potentials (EP/ERP), and pharmaco-EEG can provide a physiological endpoint that may be used to facilitate drug discovery, optimize lead or candidate compound selection, as well as afford patient stratification and decisions in clinical trials. Most important ones are well-established and emerging EEG analytic approaches that are currently being integrated from drug discovery programs throughout preclinical development and clinical trials. Also there is a significant use of EEG in the drug development process in the context of a number of major disorders such as Alzheimer's disease (AD), schizophrenia, depression, attention deficit hyperactivity disorder (ADHD), epilepsy and pain. Selection and validation of EEG endpoints that provide a set of biomarkers bridging preclinical and clinical programs seem to be another important challenge in the neuroscience world.

There have been detailed studies about introduction of wavelets and adaptive approximations of EEG which has been an important tool in neuroscience and clinical neurophysiology. Time-frequency solutions to several standard research and clinical problems, encountered in analysis of evoked potentials, sleep EEG, epileptic activities and pharmaco-EEG are studied and based on those results it is concluded that the matching pursuit algorithm provides a unified parameterization of EEG, applicable in a variety of experimental and clinical setups. Recently emerging dynamic imaging techniques like fMRI and PET offer complementary information on brain's functioning. They include significantly lower time resolution, high cost and invasiveness. However they are often preferred for the straightforward interpretability. On the contrary, visual interpretation of EEG is a difficult, tedious and complicated task which would contain a significant subjective factor. EEG interpretation would always have a personal approach.

There have been studies about statistical methods to estimate treatment effects from multichannel electroencephalography (EEG) data in clinical trials. The most common objective for analyzing the EEG data in a pharmaceutical clinical trial is to detect or estimate the difference between the change induced in EEG by the test drug and that introduced by placebo, which is called EEG treatment effect. Clinical trials were used as example datasets, and drug effect estimates were obtained and eventually the smoothed methods do require much more computation. However, with cheap computational resources increasingly available, downside of the methods will become less and less an obstacle.

Settings and objectives of the EEG, other electrophysiological and neuroimaging in trials will be exemplified and summarized below to be able to discuss the relevant ethical obstacles or requirements for ethically justified, properly designed clinical trials where human subjects are protected while electrophysiology measures are progressively more used to aid diagnosis and treatment in psychiatry.

Arnold O. reports that in a double-blind, placebo-controlled crossover study, the effects of S-adenosyl-L-methionine (SAMe) on brain function measures of 12 normal elderly volunteers (6m/6f, aged 57-73 years, Mean: 61 years) were investigated by means of EEG mapping and psychometry. QEEG data demonstrated significant central effects of SAMe as compared with placebo after acute, subacute and superimposed drug administration of both the nutraceutical and pharmaceutical dose. Psychometric tests generally demonstrated a lack of differences between SAMe and placebo, which reflects a good tolerability of the drug in elderly patients. A vast number of works has described the use of qEEG to predict the effects of pharmaceutical agents as well as to classify disease states. The activity of a number of subcortical neurotransmitter systems from several brain regions outside the thalamus is supported neurobiological that can directly impact cortical activity patterns. These neurotransmitter systems are generally targets of pharmacological intervention or participate in neurological disease states. In many clinical trials, EEG measures of cortical activity are proposed to have the potential to be an extremely powerful surrogate biomarker of depression that is translatable across species. Neurobiological etiology of schizophrenia is poorly understood. Two theories such as abnormal development of cortical networks and impaired sensory information processing are supported by the abnormalities in EEG frequency band power and measures of 'sensory gating'. Although EP/ERP based approaches are also very promising as translational biomarkers of schizophrenia, bridging the gap between preclinical and clinical findings remains challenging. EEG signals recorded from the brain can be modulated by somatosensory signals stimulated in peripheral nerves. Those evoked potentials are carried to the brain and in response to painful stimuli are processed by averaging to extract the first negative (N1) and second positive (P2) components. In Alzheimer's disease, outside of impaired cognitive functions, neurobiological changes associated with AD progression can additionally present as altered physiological functions including sleep patterns, changes in EEG activity (spectral shifts) and EP / ERP responses, as well as an increase in epileptiform and/ or seizure activity. Over the past several decades there has been considerable effort in exploring the utility of polisomnography, qEEG, and EP/ ERP measures as useful clinical markers of early disease or progression biomarkers of AD. Seizure activity and/or epileptiform discharges as measured by EEG have the additional promise as a novel biomarker for AD and such EEG based measures of neurological function offer a number of translatable, physiological endpoints that are likely indicative of disease progression in both Alzheimer's Disease patients and animal models.

EEG measures in normal volunteering subjects can initially provide evidence of CNS penetration and drug-target engagement. For example, compound classes or families have been shown to exhibit a unique electrophysiological signature. (In pharmaco-EEG trials). Nonetheless, the evoked potential endpoints are important to facilitate the early decision making process around new candidate advancement in the clinic.

Determinants of cortical activity through EEG measures permit a generic biomarker strategy with potential for broad utility across multiple CNS disorders. An aggregate of biomarkers including EEG/ERP measures will be needed to both fully classify individual cognitive disorders as well as predict the therapeutic actions of compound families. Imaging methods such as Positron emission tomography (PET), functional Magnetic Resonance Imaging (fMRI) and Magnetoencephalography (MEG) may also prove to be an important adjunct to accurately and precisely identify changes in neurological function. MEG may offer similar promise as EEG but is still emerging.

Avakian et al reports that, fifty-four patients with partial epilepsy (age 18-50 years, 26 males and 28 females, illness duration from 6 months to 18 years) have been examined. Idiopathic epilepsy was diagnosed in 7 patients, symptomatic in 36, cryptogenic in 11. The control group comprised 22 sex- and age-matched individuals. All the patients underwent computerized EEG and pharmaco-EEG testing, MRI or CT of the brain. An antioxidant therapeutic course was conducted during 30 days on the background of the basic anticonvulsive therapy with carbamazepine. As a result, EEG may be considered as a favorable prognostic factor, which reduces probability of the secondary generalization of partial epileptic seizures.

Yoshimura et al. carried out a pharmaco-EEG study. The rationale was that both psychotropic drugs and mental disorders have typical signatures in qEEG. Previous studies had found that some psychotropic drugs had EEG effects opposite to the EEG effects of the mental disorders treated with these drugs. (Key-lock principle)They performed a placebo-controlled pharmaco-EEG study on conventional and atypical antipsychotics in healthy volunteers. This study was reported to be conducted in accordance with the Declaration of Helsinki (1964), and approved by the institutional ethical review board. All subjects participated voluntarily after being fully informed about the study and having given their written consent and each subject was paid an amount equivalent to approximately 2700.00 USD for the entire experiment. Eventually, the increased microstate duration under perospirone and haloperidol was opposite to effects previously reported in schizophrenic patients, suggesting a key-lock mechanism. The opposite centroid changes induced by olanzapine and quetiapine compared to haloperidol might characterize the difference between conventional and atypical antipsychotics.

Price et al. accomplished a study that uses an EEG-dependent technique as a means to enhance the efficacy of rTMS in the treatment of depression and that the use of EEG-based TMS stimuli might be more feasible in an rTMS clinical trial in treatment resistant depression. Forty-four patients with treatment-refractory major depression were treated in a randomized, double-blind, 4-week trial, with two different rTMS stimulus timing techniques. Standard rTMS utilizing 10-Hz stimuli where interactive rTMS applied individual stimuli in response to a selected pattern of background EEG activity analyzed in real time. The interactive technique showed a greater clinical effect than the standard. The interactive technique was concluded to have the potential to refine the rTMS methodology and to enhance efficacy in the treatment of depression.

Loss et al emphasize that many of the monitors that are increasingly used to titrate sedation and avoid awareness during anesthesia are based on EEG collected from large adult reference populations and not pediatric populations. They hypothesized that EEG patterns in children would be different from those ty4previously reported in adults. This was planned as a prospective observational study and was approved by IRB and informed written consent was obtained. Patients were randomized to receive maintenance anesthesia with isoflurane or sevoflurane and EEG data collection included at least 10 min at steady-state maintenance anesthesia. The EEG was recorded continuously through emergence until extubation.37 children between ages of 22 days-3.6 years) completed the study. There were anesthetic-specific and concentration-dependent EEG effects in children. Depth –of-anesthesia monitors that utilize EEGs of adult reference populations may not be appropriate for use in children.

Other clinical trials like measurements of vagus nerve stimulation (rTMS) in the treatment of depression comparing with neurobiological effects measured with neuroimaging (fTMI), biochemical and electrophysiology (EEG) approaches have enlightened various mechanisms. Integrative processing between the different sensory modalities and the neuronal mechanisms underlying the reaction time facilitation effect has been investigated by Senkowski et al. measuring oscillatory beta activity. It has been concluded that the association between oscillatory beta activity and integrative multisensory processing is directly linked to multisensory reaction time facilitation effects. Subjects that were chosen pressed buttons to indicate the appearance of any stimulation in a stream of auditory, visual or multisensory stimulus and measured beta oscillations were evaluated. Electrophysiology trials promising in diagnostic and treatment tool for neurological disorders like diabetic polyneuropathy, other neuromuscular diseases, and neurophysiologic measures as markers of progression of amyotrophic lateral sclerosis have been developing over the past decade, as well. Roche Neuropathy Study Group evaluated 253 normal subjects and 1345 patients with mild DPN at 60 international centers. All waveforms, distances and calibration signals were reviewed in a blinded fashion by two electromyographic techniques. Neurophysiologic evaluation will permit inferences of mechanism of therapeutic action not only for DPN but also for amyotrophic lateral sclerosis.

As exemplified in section 1.7, Kayran et al carried out a randomized, blind study to assess the efficacy of EEG Biofeedback (Neurofeedback) in patients with fibromyalgia syndrome18 patients received twenty sessions of NFB-sensory motor rhythm (SMR) treatment (NFM group) during 4 weeks, and 18 patients were given 10 mg per day escilopram treatment (control group) for 8 weeks. Therapeutic efficacy of NFB was found to begin at 2nd week and reached to a maximum effect at 4th week. Improvements in SSRI treatment were also detected to begin at 2nd week but reached to a maximum effect at 8th week. No statistically significant changes were noted regarding mean amplitudes of EEG rhythms. However, theta/SMR ratio showed a significant decrease at 4th week compared to baseline in the NFB group. These data supported the efficacy of NFB as a treatment for pain, psychological symptoms and impaired quality of life associated with fibromyalgia. This study indicated that NBF procedure cannot be put in the first line treatment procedure.

Besides the literature examples, I wished to sum up the clinical trials of the *first* joint ECNS / ISBET /ISNIP conference organized in September 2010 in Istanbul, with respect to general principles and ethical arguments: Repetitive TMS (rTMS) trials were usually used against chronic pain and depression stimulating prefrontal and dorsolateral cortex and against pain in fibromyalgia as well. It did not prove to be affective against panic disorder. rTMS / fMRI studies were also used for the same purpose. Neurofeedback trials using EEG, qEEG for depression, ADHD, substance abuse, performance anxiety, rehabilitating cognitive performance during mild traumatic brain injury, behavioral and cognitive peculiarities in children were commonly used. "EEG Statistical Parametric Mapping of the First Year of Life" was a very interesting trial accomplished in 100 normal infant subjects, from 1 to 12 months of age. Also electrophysiology trials were used to solve the interrelated mechanisms of the brain such as: "Is function predetermined by anatomical connections?" PET and fMRI trials were usually accomplished for the diagnosis of

Alzheimer's Disease to further detect the neurobiological changes. EEG readings and multimodal neuroimaging studies have been reported to give strong clues about the unsolved mechanisms of schizophrenia. In some studies, EEG-fMRI data are recorded simultaneously from healthy volunteers to make an approach to steady-state evoked responses of the brain and retention phase of short-term memory.

After recording EEG traces in 1920s, magnetoencephalography (MEG) was developed towards the end of 1960s. MEG measures magnetic field strength of a field occurring with a 90 degree angle to the electrical current, while it is more successful in localizing the source of neuronal activity, more precise in localizing biomagnetic foci in subcortical regions of the brain and realtime 3D recordings can be recorded. A combined use of MEG MRI enables to show the magnetic activity distribution in the brain or magnetic source localization such as epileptic foci. In a study where epileptic activity is present in one subgroup of schizophrenic patients, the relationship between schizophrenia and epilepsy is investigated with EEG and MEG and MEG was successful in localizing epileptic foci.

As a consensus, human brain is organized according to two fundamental principles, functional segregation and functional integration. Segregation is the regional differentiation of the cerebral cortex into specialized modules and integration denotes the inter-regional connectivity of anatomical, functional and effective connectivity. With respect to the mentioned concepts, in combination with electrical and fMRI brain imaging techniques, brain electrical activity mapping is an appropriate and useful tool for investigating sensory and cognitive functions of the human central nervous system.

Experiences from Institutional Review Boards about EEG trials in Turkey

It is known that EEG as a tool of diagnostic and treatment procedures has a defined role in psychiatry patients. It is mostly not risky and harmless. Sometimes time concern and the physical restrictions are burden for the patients. However, EEG can very easily be modified in applications and used on irrelevant patients just for research purposes or replace drug therapy. As an example, we had some experience of researches offering EEG applications after bypass surgery for the purpose of detecting some functions of the brain to observe the efficiency of blood circulation. However, according to our experience, when it is used out of the range of accepted measures and definitions, it becomes a clinical trial and if appropriate informed consent is not taken, patients may become anxious and prognosis might become worse. Besides, if economic parameters are not monitored properly, then patients might be under a heavy burden.

From theory to practice

In Turkey, we have come through a long way with the concept of informed consent in clinical trials, ethics committees (IRBs), health care professionals and public, as the country's talks with European Union is continuing. However, there are still fundamental obstacles about clinical trials and informed consent.

Necessity and safety of the trials in Turkey

Lately, a positive report has been observed about healthy human subjects joining clinical trials in Turkey. The trial was roughly about the comparing the efficiency of bioequivalent drugs in healthy human subjects. If subjects justified the prerequisite conditions, they were accepted for the trial and were required to sign the informed consent form. Before, it was reported that only a small number of people volunteered for such studies but now the number reached 12000 in one of the research centers. The center mentioned that the real incentive was money. There has always been an ambiguity about the relatively new concept .informed consent. in clinical trials in Turkey. There have been very negative responses about giving consent to swine flu vaccination in Turkey in 2009-2010. Although rates of vaccination against regular seasonal flu and pneumonia were quite normal, few people gave consent for swine flu vaccination and even parents for elementary school students. The main reason is emphasized was a lack of confidence in the necessity and safety of the trial and a very obscure informed consent process.

A small local study from Turkey

To understand the attitudes of randomized healthy people towards clinical trials and informed consent process, we carried out a small qualitative research among 200 healthy volunteering subjects above 18 years of age in a small town in a the most populous city of Turkey (Istanbul). Five questions were asked and subjects wrote down their ideas. No interview took place. The inclusion criteria of the subjects were to be healthy and not to be hospitalized when they took place in the study, to volunteer to answer the questions and to be competent.

The questions were:

1. *What is clinical research?*
2. *Would you like to join a clinical research project? Would you demand to get paid?*
3. *How would you know if the clinical trial has risks or benefits for your life?*
4. *Do you understand the informed consent forms? How do you feel when you read them?*
5. *Are you familiar with the idea from your experience or environment that physicians explain clearly if they will carry on a research project or apply conventional treatment when you are admitted as a patient?*

Data were evaluated with descriptive statistics and were assessed bu simple percentage calculation.

Results:

90% of the participants did not clearly realize what a clinical trial was, by experience. 95% did not like very long informed consent forms. They complained that they did not understand clearly what was written on them and those forms made them feel nervous and they got scared of the procedure. 80% declared that they would not prefer to get involved in a research project unless it was very necessary when they were sick or when there was not any other alternative. They just mentioned by assumption that if they would join as healthy subjects they would like to be paid and this would be possible only with the condition of having minimum risk. 90 % of participants were not familiar of the idea of the physician's explaining them or somebody from their environment that they would be included in a safe trial.

The answers did not have a cumulative percentage accumulation according to the demographic and educational background of the patients.

Around 2 % of the participants could not successfully answer some questions, those questions being different for every participating individual. Those will be deliberated later in the discussion section.

So far, we might conclude that many research projects and clinical trials are being carried out by a variety of disciplines like neuropsychiatry, neurophysiology etc. about EEG, comparative methods like fMRI, neuroimaging and brain functions all around the world. Although there are differences between the perspectives of different countries in handling the ethical issues in clinical trials, we observe that ethical justification and informed consent is inevitable and there is an ongoing debate about the topic in different disciplines and cultures.

There are also some common shared and some culture dependent facts and ethical discussion points about the above mentioned clinical trials in Turkey.

What makes clinical research ethical?

Emanuel from NIH reports that

- Informed consent
- IRB review
- Compliance with Nuremberg Code, Declaration of Helsinki, and Belmont Report or other relevant guidelines
- Compliance with national legislation protecting human subjects
- Or all of the above make clinical research ethical.

Clinical research develops generalizable knowledge that improves health or increases understanding. People who participate in clinical research are a means to securing that generalizable knowledge. Subjects in trials can be exploited, that is be used for the benefits of others. Ethical requirements for clinical research are meant to minimize the possibility of exploitation. All ethical guidelines developed in response to a problem, respond to the controversy and do not provide a systematic ethical framework. Frequently they are incomplete and also might contradict each other. In practice eight ethical requirements are proposed to be justified in order as guidelines would never be enough and complete for a review process:

- Collaborative partnership
- Social Value
- Scientific validity
- Fair subject selection
- Favorable risk-benefit ratio
- Independent review
- Informed consent
- Respect for human subjects

DISCUSSION

The EEG has been used for many purposes besides the conventional uses of clinical diagnosis and conventional cognitive neuroscience. Long-term EEG recordings in epilepsy patients are used for seizure prediction. Neurofeedback remains an important extension, and in its most advanced form is also attempted as the basis of brain computer interfaces.

Current neuroscience research projects are using EEG and other electrophysiological measures such as EEG/ERP, pharmaco-EEG, MEG, polysomnography or other techniques such as fMRI, TMS or PET to answer questions relevant to better care of patients in the future with unknown mechanisms of disease. Although each technique proposes a different research setting and while this process is going on with the enthusiasm of hardworking researchers, we are still concerned about some commonly observed ethical problems such as mis-un-true informed consent, problems of fair subject selection, money's role in trials etc.

After the first ECNS / ISBET / ISNIP Joint Meeting that was organized between September 14-18, 2010 in Istanbul / Turkey with participants from many different countries and from a variety of disciplines, we had observed that neuroscience is beginning to develop very rapidly through various research projects bringing many ethical issues about human subjects to stage. We observed that every country tries to handle the ethical issues according to their very specific conditions on a culture dependent way and according to their Institutional Review Board review protocol and regulations although guidelines regarding research consent are well known and widely available.

When the presentations were reviewed, very little was claimed about informed consent and how the trial was planned in terms of protecting human subjects although the attitude differed from one project to another and from one center to another. Also reviewed clinical trial examples above show the same pattern while some researchers claiming about informed consent in their articles, some do not. However, when we evaluated the answers of researchers to the questions, we could easily conclude that everybody was aware of the ethical issues and but preferred to handle them in a different manner for a variety of reasons. We do not want to name every researcher and country here specifically since the correspondence was an oral conversation, permission was not taken and it is not our primary concern. However, we still feel the responsibility to report that, just for the sake of the difficulty in the informed consent process, some researchers bypassed it, or carried out the trial without control group subjects, or did not inform the subjects about the clinical trial but would present the trial as a conventional treatment to the patients while some researchers definitely preferred a very proper protocol in planning the trial considering the safety of human subjects and informing them in a proper way. Participants had agreed that there was not a network worldwide or an efficient communication and standards between the functioning IRBs and enforced legislations although a long way had been completed by the efforts of professionals and societies.

I won't discuss in this book unethical researches or professionals that are deliberately exploiting human subjects or patients such as the ever profiteering drug industry, the ever loosening professional standards of the physician and the standing and expectations from the state health authorities although we know that they exist. Those situations are reported occasionally and the precautions are straight forward such as proper control mechanisms and punishment. I will discuss the issues that are unwanted, unknown, results of unawareness and deteriorate clinical trials' settings and happens although it was never intended so. Systematic ethical requirements or approaches are suggested in practice.

Mental health professionals or researchers might have variety unethical characteristics even if they prefer or respect or believe to be ethical such as "rationalize actions that are often unrecognized as self-serving", "Are ignorant or misinformed regarding the ethical standards of their profession", "Usually behave competently, ethically, and with good awareness, but 'slip' by losing sight of a goal or becoming momentarily distracted," "suffer from burnout or other emotional impairment." Besides those very possible unethical characteristics of the professionals or researchers, there are specific characteristics and important issues about clinical trials that would cause unethical approach to human subjects.

We know that EEG as an electrophysiological measure of diagnostic and treatment procedures has a defined conventional role in psychiatry or neurology but also a promising role in clinical trials for future patients. The inexpensive hardware, along with new signal processing technologies that have appeared in the past 10 years has rendered EEG technology extremely accessible. EEG's noninvasive nature, simple implementation and relatively cheap operational cost have helped to revitalize to attraction among pharmaceutical companies. EEG has recently more and more been seen as a critical modality in clinical trials. As of September 2009, over 320 studies involving EEG have been registered with 'clinicaltrials.gov' a website logging clinical trials conducted in the United States and around the world.

As a technique, it is mostly not risky and harmless. Sometimes time concern and the physical restrictions are burden for the patients especially when recorded after having had a serious surgery such as bypass. However, EEG can very easily be modified in applications and used on irrelevant patients just for research purposes without being properly informed or replace drug therapy such as some of the neurofeedback trials again without proper information and with some hope instead. However, when it is used out of the range of accepted measures and definitions, it becomes a clinical trial and if appropriate "informed consent" is not taken, patients may become anxious about their expectations or outcomes and prognosis of their disease state might be affected in a negative way. Besides, if economic parameters are not monitored properly, then patients might be under a heavy burden. Characteristic methods of clinical trials are randomization, blinding, placebo, comparing with different patient control groups with different doses of stimulations or drug therapies (informed consent being a serious problem) or healthy volunteering subjects paid as an incentive and common aim is always to minimize bias and respect diversity in designing and implementing research. Those methods would support a proper methodology, reliable and valid data but would replace informed consent and autonomy in a questionable state at the same time.

Pharmaco-EEG trials have some other ethical concerns. As Silvana discusses, multi-dose, placebo-controlled studies with multiple pre- and post-drug measurements are to be used to compensate for spontaneous or experimentally induced biases. So, pharmaco-EEG clinical trials are not as straight forward as trials of fast developing techniques for functional brain imaging such as fMRI, TMS or NFB. These point out that because of limitations of a correct experimental setting and correct management of interactions with human subjects, one of which is informed consent and others are fair subject selection and scientific validity, are very important in pharmaco-EEG clinical trials to reduce the variability in electrophysiological changes attributable to drug. On the other hand, large-scale studies have high costs. Healthy subjects used in the comparison of different dosage of anti-psychotic drugs that need to be paid is another issue for concern for fair subject selection. For pharmaco-EEG studies, important issues of ethics to be implemented might be grouped as:

1. Research must be conducted in a methodologically rigorous manner that is practically feasible,
2. To be ethical the research must produce reliable and valid data that can be interpreted,
3. Invalid research includes underpowered studies, studies with biased endpoints, instruments, or statistical tests, and studies that cannot enroll sufficient subjects,
4. Convenient groups should not be selected,
5. Higher risk is a reason to exclude certain groups,

6. Clinical research must be conducted in a manner consistent with the standards of clinical practice.
7. Consider physical, psychological, social, and economic benefits to the individual.
8. Informed consent ensures individuals decide whether they enroll in research and whether research fits with their own values, interests, and goals.

Normal volunteers participate in pharmaco-EEG studies as well as other EEG and neuroscience trials sometimes double-blind, placebo-controlled and randomized. Studies are performed in accordance with the relevant guidelines of the Declaration of Helsinki, protocols are approved by IRBs and subjects are paid. Is money an incentive in research? Or are there other motives such as curiosity, altruism, contributing to science, sensation seeking? How do consideration of other factors such as risk, time and inconvenience contribute in participation? What might be the barriers for participation? Money is considered to be an incentive for healthy volunteers but not so in patient participants of research. Risk assessment, minimizing risk, time, inconvenience, informed consent and amount of money to be paid should be reviewed by IRBs. Ethical concerns about paying would be a skewed sample as money would be more attractive to lower income participants, coercion and undue inducement or influence. Successfully and ethically recruiting the right number and type of participants may be facilitated by understanding the reasons why people participate, incentives for participation and barriers to participation.

EEG, pharmaco-EEG or other neuroscience clinical trials when applied to children subjects who cannot consent, or to mentally impaired, then we must be sure research fits with their interests. Prospect of benefit interventions offer a chance of clinical benefit that is at least as good as clinical care, such as pharmaco-EEG trial of phase three drug studies. Non beneficial interventions pose risks to pediatric subjects and do not offer a chance for clinical benefit such as research blood draws included in phase three studies. This can be acceptable only when risks are acceptable and the intervention has the potential to collect valuable information that justifies the risks the subjects face.

EEG was the only objective parameter for a long time providing information on brain's function. Recently emerging dynamic imaging techniques like fMRI and PET offer complementary information on brain's functioning as we have reviewed before. Their drawbacks as trial settings include significantly lower time resolution, high cost and invasiveness with relevance to the ethical challenge of minimal risk. Nevertheless, in spite of these drawbacks, they are often preferred to the straightforward interpretability. Then physical, psychological, social and economic risks should be evaluated for the likelihood of harm and risks should be identified, assessed and minimized.

Every trial has a different setting, certain scientific limitations and benefits. However, whatever the research type is and since the guidelines are never enough in practice as we have discussed before, we need to apply the eight ethical requirements that justify that research is ethical in practice in common. Rosenstein from University of North Caroline (UNC) reports that research with decisionally impaired adults is different than medical care and is up to the "Informed Consent Requirements" designated by the legislations that deals with the protection of human subjects. Informed consent ensures individuals decide whether they enroll in research and whether research fits with their own values, interests, and goals. Neuro Feed Back studies if they replace drug therapies give unjustified hope and proposed as conventional therapeutic tools to patients with apparent conflicts of interest with uninformed consent or straightforward rTMS studies are done without proper control groups and misinformed consent then ethical obstacles are created.

So far, we might conclude that many research projects and clinical trials are being carried out by a variety of disciplines like neuropsychiatry, neurophysiology etc. about EEG, pharmaco-EEG, TMS, PET, MEG, comparative methods like fMRI, neuroimaging and brain functions. Although there are differences between the perspectives of different countries in handling the ethical issues in clinical trials, we observe that a proper risk assessment, fair subject selection, ethical justification and informed consent is inevitable. Eight ethical requirements should be justified in practice to prevent ethical obstacles and to protect human subjects. There is an ongoing debate about the topic in different disciplines and cultures and institutions try to manage them by Institutional Review Boards.

Reidar from National Institute of Health of USA emphasizes that common complaints for IRBs are that members are overworked, there might be delay in review of protocols and some of this can be resolved by appropriate procedures like expedited review and qualification requirement of membership. Rosenstein from UNC reports that research with decisionally impaired adults is different from medical care and is up to the Informed Consent Requirements designated by 45 CFR Part 46 that deals with the protection of human subjects. Emanuel emphasizes that besides the regulation, there are other ethical requirements that are universal and not culture dependent and that make clinical research ethical.

According to Arikan, Turkish subjects in psychiatry tend to either take a totally submissive position or show total rage during the informed consent procedure; yet they rarely ask for alternatives or question details. Informed consent has not been part of routine clinical practice until recent years and both researchers and subjects seem yet to be unfamiliar with the process. These comments comply with our research results.

Oguz from Turkey reports that informed consent that is related to personal autonomy is a Western setting. In developing countries the autonomy is rather collective and mainly based on previous experiences, beliefs and traditions. This difference puts the whole process of informed consent in developing countries in question.

Arikan discusses that when too much information is given to the patient or the family in Turkey, it might lead to suspicion and disbelief in Turkish society. The process rapidly enhances a feeling of extraordinariness and some kind of paranoid thinking since it has not been part of the routine in the standard medical care in Turkey until recent times.

There is an ongoing debate about the topic in different disciplines and cultures and institutions try to manage them by IRBs.

LAST WORD

We might conclude that many research projects and clinical trials are being carried out by a variety of disciplines like neuropsychiatry, neurophysiology etc. about EEG, pharmaco-EEG, TMS, PET, MEG, comparative methods like fMRI, neuroimaging and brain functions. Although there are differences between the perspectives of different countries in handling the ethical issues in clinical trials, we observe that a proper risk assessment, fair subject selection, ethical justification and informed consent are inevitable. Eight ethical requirements should be justified in practice to prevent ethical obstacles and to protect human subjects.

However, Turkish society is evolving and the government is progressively having more open institutions. In terms of process and the future, physicians are also changing their traditional and culture-dominated paternalistic role. Informed consent is trying to establish and maintain its role in patient-physician relationship.

My new expression in clinical trials would be **"Mis-Un-True"** Informed Consent and it seems to take place as an ethical challenge. My impression as to the application of this new concept in clinical trials might have the danger or possibility of, currently, either of *"misinformed consent"*, *"uninformed consent"* or *"true informed consent"*, depending on the conditions. Informed consent still needs a good evaluation and formulation considering the researchers' responsibilities and subjects' protection considering cultural elements in every society.

Although there are difficulties for a variety of reasons we have mentioned above, informed consent is inevitable and essential ethical requirement in patient-physician relationship in clinical trials of any kind.

From an objective viewpoint; uninformed consent or misinformed consent is not efficient and acceptable in any situation, especially in trials. A proper "Informed Consent" will be the indicator of a successful clinical trial all around the world. A

38

common ground or a better sharing network composed of comprehensive professionals and ethicists seems necessary and promising for the future process of trials in a variety of disciplines of neuroscience and psychiatry.

Practically speaking, since EEG and its derivatives cannot be claimed that they have the absolute value of diagnosis, treatment and follow up, any information given to the patients must be stressed in this regard. Otherwise, it would be a good example of *mis-un-true* informed consent.

REFERENCES

Abou-Khalil B, Musilus, K.E. (2006) Atlas of EEG & Seizure Semiology. Elsevier.

Anderson J. (2005) Cognitive Psychology and its Implications, 6th Ed., Worth Publishers, New York, NY, p: 17.

Andre-Obedia N, Merhens P, Lelekov-Boissard et al.(2014) Is life better after motor cortex stimulation for pain control? Results at long-term and their prediction by preoperative rTMS. Pain Physician. 17(1):53-62.

Arezzo JC. (1999) New developments in the diagnosis of diabetic neuropathy. Am J Med; 107 (2B): 9S-16S.

Arikan K. (2010) Turkish Experience of Ethics in Clinical Research: A Psychiatrist's Perspective. in: Dogan H, Lie R. (eds) Proceedings of International Workshop on Advanced Clinical Research Ethics. NIH, Precision Printing, UK. 189-191.

Arnold O, Saletu B, Anderer P. et al. (2005) Double-blind, placebo-controlled pharmacodynamic studies with a nutraceutical and a pharmaceutical dose of ademetionine (SAMe) in elderly subjects, utilizing EEG mapping and psychometry. European Neuropsychopharmacology. 15: 533-543.

Avakian GK, Ryzhova MV, Badalian OL et al. (2005) Use of a 3-oxypiridine antioxidant in combined therapy of patients with partial epilepsy. Nevrol Psikhiatr im SS Korsakova. 105 (6): 21-5.

Carvalto M. Ohio A. Dengler R. Hecht M. et al. (2005) Neurophysiologic measures in amyotrophic lateral sclerosis: markers of progression in clinical trials. Motor Neuron Disord. 6 (1):17-28.

Dogan H. (2010) Critical Role of Informed Consent in Turkish Society in Clinical Trials. In: Dogan H, Lie R. (Eds) Proceedings of International Workshop on Advanced Clinical Research Ethics. NIH, Precision Printing, UK. 164-168.

Dogan H. et al. (2015) Quality and extent of informed consent for invasive procedures: a pilot study at the institutional level in Turkey. Int J Qual in Health Care. 27(1), 46-51.

Dogan H. (2012) Clinical Trials: The physician with the Hat of a Researcher. J. of Med Ethics, Law and History. 20(2), 115-120.

Dogan H. (2011) Mis-Un-True Informed Consent: A Brief Report from Turkey and a comparative study about "Ethics in Clinical Trialsof EEG" in Psychiatry. EJAIB. 21(6), 212-217.

Donald S. (2010) Important Issues about Clinical Research. In: Dogan H. Transition to Clinical Ethics. Istanbul. 114-124.

Durka JP. (2003) from wavelets to adaptive approximations: time-Frequency parametrization of EEG. Biomed Eng Online. 2(1):1-12. (Published online 9 January 6. Doi: 1011861475-925x-2-1.

Emanuel Z. (2010) What Makes Clinical Research Ethical? In: Dogan H, Lie R. (Eds) Proceedings of International Workshop on Advanced Clinical Research Ethics. NIH, Precision Printing, UK. 12-22.

ECNS / ISBET / ISNIP Joint Meeting (2010). Abstract Booklet. Istanbul September 14-18, 2010 :8,9,13-19,21-25,27-30,32-34,39-41,43-46.

Galdirisi S. (2006) Pharmaco-EEG at a Crossroads.Clinical EEG and Neuroscience. 37(2): 60.

Galderisi S, Sannite WG. (2006) Pharmaco-EEG: A History of Progress and a Missed Opportunity. Clinical EEG and Neuroscience.37 (2): 61-65.

Grady C. (2010) Payment and incentives. In: Dogan H, Lie R. (Eds) Proceedings of International Workshop on Advanced Clinical Research Ethics. NIH, Precision Printing, UK. 68-73.

Grimm S, Bajbouj M. (2010) Efficacy of vagus nerve stimulation in the treatment of depression. Expert Rev Neurother. 10(1):87-92.

Junshui M. Shubing W, Richard R, Vladimir S. (2010) Statistical methods to estimate treatment effects from multichannel electroencephalography (EEG) data in clinical trials. Journal of Neuroscience Methods. 190: 248-257.

Kaufman P, O'Rourke PP. (2015) Central Institutional Review Board Review for an academic trial network. Academic Med. Mar; 90(3):321-3. Doi:10.1097/ACM.0000000000000562.

Kayran S, Dursun E, Dursun N et al. (2010). Karamürsel S. Neurofeedback Intervention in Fibromyalgia Syndrome; a Randomized, Controlled, Rater Blind Clinical Trial. Appl Psychophysiol Biofeedback.

Koocher Gerald P, Keith-Spiegel Patricia. (2008) Ethics in Psychology and the Mental Health Professions. (Eds). 3rd Edition. Oxford University Press. 8-12.

Lally PJ, Pauliah S, Montaldo P. et al. (2015) Magnetis Resonance Biomarkers in Neonatal Encephalopaty (MARBLE): a prospoective multicountry study. BMJ Open. 30:5 (9) e008912 doi: 10.1136bmjopen.

Leiser CS, Dunlop J, Bowlby MR, Devillbiss DM. (2010) Aligning strategies for using EEG as a surrogate biomarker: A review of preclinical and clinical research. Biochem Pharmacol. In press: 1-14 Doi: 10.1016/j.bcp.2010.10.002.

Lie R. Organization of Ethics Review. (2010) In: Dogan H, Lie R. (Eds) Proceedings of International Workshop on Advanced Clinical Research Ethics. NIH, Precision Printing, UK: 34-36.

LoSS, Sobol JB, Mallavaram N, Carsan M. et al. (2009) Anesthetic-specific electroencephalographic patterns during emergence from sevoflurane and isoflurane in infants and children. Pediatr Anaesth. 19(12): 1157–65.

Matthew JB, Jonathan RW, Claire MS, Johanna MZ et al. (2010) Changes in brain network activity during working memory tasks: A magnetoencephalography study. Neuroimage.1-11.

Niedermeyer E. and da Silva F.L. (2007) Electroencephalography: Basic Principles, Clinical Applications, and Related Fields. Lippincott Williams & Wilkins.

Oguz NY. (2003) Research ethics committees in developing countries and informed consent: With special reference to Turkey. Journal of Laboratory and Clinical Medicine. 141: 292-296.

Price GW, Lee JN, Garvey CA, Gibson N. (2010) The use of background EEG activity to determine stimulus timing as a means of improving rTMS efficacy in the treatment of depression. Brain Stimul. 3(3):140-52.

Richard K. Olney MD. (1998) Neurophysiologic Evaluation and Clinical Trials for Neuromuscular Diseases. Muscle Nerve. 21:1365-1367.

Rosenstein D. (2010) Informed Consent and Research with Decisionally Impaired Adults. In: Dogan H, Lie R. (Eds) Proceedings of International Workshop on Advanced Clinical Research Ethics. NIH, Precision Printing, UK. 44-52.

Schicktanz S, Schweda M, Ballenger JF. (2014).Before it is too late: professional responsibilities in late-onset Alzheimer's research and pre-symptomatic prediction. Front Hum Neurosci. 20; 8:921. Doi: 10.3389/fnhum.

Senkowski D, Malholm S, Ramitrez M and Foxe J. (2010) Oscillatory Beta Activity Predicts Response Speed during a Multisensory Audiovisual Reaction Time Task: A High-Density Electrical Mapping Study. Oxford Journals. Life Sciences and Medicine. Cerebral Cortex 16 (11): 1556-1565.

Twelve- thousand people volunteered to be human subjects in a clinical trial.(2009) Milliyet Nationwide Newspaper 20. 1-2.

Underwood E. (2015). NEUROSCIENCE. Brain Implant Trials Raise Ethical Concerns. Science. 348 (6240): 1186-7. Doi: 10.1126/science.348.6240.1186.

Wendler D. Research on Children: Risk Assessments. (2010) In: Dogan H, Lie R. (Eds) Proceedings of International Workshop on Advanced Clinical Research Ethics. NIH, Precision Printing UK. 60-67.

Yazıcı H. (2007) Use and Abuse of the Controlled Clinical Trial. Bulletin of the NYU Hospital for Joint Diseases. 65(2):132-4.

Yoshimura M, Koenig T, Irisawa S, Isotani T, Yamaha K et al. (2007) A Paharmaco-EEG study on antipsychotic drugs in healthy volunteers. Psychopharmacology. 191: 995-1004.

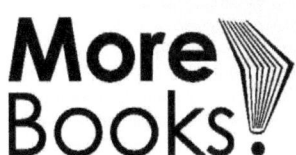
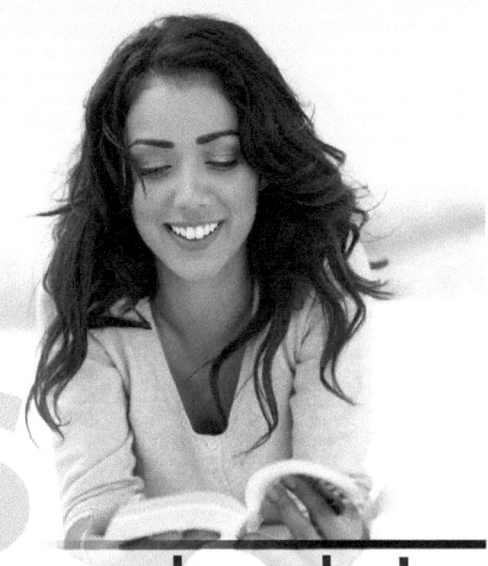
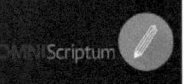

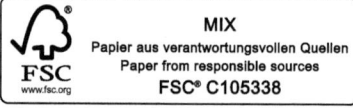
Printed by Books on Demand GmbH, Norderstedt / Germany